CU00691357

# Easy Pilates Exercises
## to
# Improve Posture

## KRISTEN FRYER

**EASY PILATES EXERCISES TO IMPROVE POSTURE is**
**© Copyright 2016 Kristen Fryer**
IntuitPilates.com

**Published by FLYING DONKEY PRESS – Placerville, CA**
FlyingDonkeyPress.com

**Cover Design by Shawn Hansen**
ShawnHansen.com

**ISBN (Paperback)**
978-1-939229-27-4

**ISBN (eBook)**
978-1-939229-28-1

**ALL RIGHTS RESERVED**
No part of this book may be reproduced or transmitted in any form whatsoever, electronic, or mechanical without express written, dated, and signed permission from Kristen Fryer.

**DISCLAIMER AND/OR LEGAL NOTICES**
All the information presented in Easy Pilates Exercises to Improve Posture (eBook) is for educational and resource purposes **only**. It is **NOT** a substitute for or an addition to any advice given to you by your Physician or Health Care Provider.

Before making any changes to your lifestyle or exercise habits and before implementing any information in this eBook you must consult your Physician.

Please understand that **you** are solely responsible for the way information in this eBook is perceived and utilized and you do so at your own risk.

In no way will **In|tu|it Pilates** or any persons associated with **In|tu|it Pilates** be held responsible for any injuries or problems that may occur due to the use of this eBook or the advice contained within.

**TO CONTACT KRISTEN FRYER**
Visit **IntuitPilates.com**, or send an e-mail to
**KristenFryer@IntuitPilates.com**

# Table of Contents

# INTRODUCTION

This little book is a result of many years of struggle. It may look like a neat little package. It may look to other people like posture and movement come easy for me. When I tell people my history many times they are shocked saying, "But you make it look so easy." It wasn't easy and it took many years, thousands of dollars and lots of study to uncover the secrets of my posture. I put together this book because I want to share what I learned. I want to help other people become comfortable in their bodies and be able to have a simple home program they can do everyday if they want.

On August 31st, 1997, (I remember the date because it's the same day that Princess Diana died) my first bout of sciatic pain hit. After dropping a stack of dishes, I crawled to the kitchen and was told to take myself to the nearby hospital. When I checked in I told the nurse I was sure my kidneys were failing because I had never experienced that level of pain. They catheterized me while I looked at images of Princess Diana's wreck on the news. I cried from my back pain and for the loss of my favorite public figure simultaneously. I was given a prescription for pain pills and told that it was a just a muscle spasm.

I went back to college and slept poorly, still tried to lift things and always felt as though my back was about to give out. I stopped dancing, running, and camping. It was all too painful. People started commenting on my poor posture, even strangers on the street! I was only 21 years old and I thought if I don't figure this out I am going to have a terrible life. I started seeing a chiropractor, which gave me some relief but the pain always came back. In the fall of 1999, my voice teacher at Berea College, Dr.

Ann Rhodes (Solberg at the time) told me I should try the Alexander Technique to improve my singing. I searched the internet and the closest teacher was a two-hour drive away.

I borrowed a car and scraped together $65 for my first lesson with the director of The Alexander Technique of Cincinnati, Vivien Schapera. After the lesson I felt so light and free and I noticed that I felt no back pain for the first time in two years. I got off the table and told her that I wanted to study the Alexander Technique when I graduated from college the next year. She looked at me like, "Are you serious?" You see, becoming an Alexander Technique teacher is a 1600-hour training that is 5 days a week 3 hours/ day and cost $20,000 out-of-pocket. At the time I was nowhere near being able to come up with that kind of money. However, against the odds I managed to move to Cincinnati that summer after graduation and got my Alexander certificate in 2002 from Vivien and her husband Neil.

The Alexander Technique changed my entire way of thinking and thus brought about big changes in my body. I went from completely unaware of my movement to noticing how tension in my big toe affected my knee. Before the technique, I was very fearful and lacked focus and discipline. Although, some of that was age, the work gave me somewhere to put my energy and allowed me to finally feel at home in my body. I hadn't felt that for a very long time it is still the greatest gift.

During my Alexander training I was introduced to the Pilates Method, which was new to Cincinnati. Vivien thought I should train to teach Pilates so I could pay for my Alexander training. The two modalities felt like total opposites and were completely confusing to me for many years: One that encourages your body to release tension and the other asking you to engage many muscle groups at once to build strength and control. I began with a quick six-month training and quickly discovered that there was more to Pilates and if I wanted to learn how to teach it well it would require a much more comprehensive training. After I graduated from Alexander school in 2002, I enrolled in the Ron Fletcher Program of Study, which required me to travel to Denver and Tucson. Ron Fletcher studied under Joseph and Clara Pilates and had also been a Martha Graham dancer. He was 82 when I met him and he taught until he died at the age of 90! I finished his program by November 2004 and have been teaching Pilates ever since.

In 2010, I started my own practice and built a lovely Pilates studio in my home, which has allowed me to be more creative in my work and to be available to my two young boys. One question

I have constantly been asked over the years is "What can I do at home to improve my posture?" this book answers that question.

## Disclaimer

This book is not pure Pilates. I have chosen to teach a routine that includes pre-Pilates concepts and a few Pilates mat exercises adapted on a foam roller. Foam Rollers did not exist in Joseph Pilates' day but many Pilates' studios teach with them now; they are a great tool for prepping the body for a full-blown Pilates workout. Pilates has been around for 115 years and it is not my intention to summarize its history. There are many great books that can take you deeper into the history of Pilates and can give you an understanding of the philosophies behind the work. My goal behind writing this is to give you a simple way to get started and see results using an inexpensive prop.

This book is not exhaustive by any means. This is one routine designed for a beginner student who is in reasonably good shape. There are many more exercises, fundamentals, props and equipment in the world of Pilates and I whole-heartedly encourage you to explore them, find a teacher and get yourself into a studio to learn more. It is a wonderful modality.

If you have osteoporosis, severe postural problems, or sciatic pain, *please check with your doctor before trying this program.* On the other side of the coin, if you are in incredible physical shape and consider yourself an advanced mover you might find this book to be too easy. However, you could use the exercises as a release after a long day at work and use the foam roller to relax built-up tension from prolonged sitting or intense manual labor.

## Why the Foam Roller?

My group classes love using the foam roller. My students often return for it every week for years. Why? Because it makes them feel so good and after they have spent many hours on a computer or sitting at a desk, they need something to release the tension. After teaching for 15 years, I have noticed problems clients were having in a group class situation, issues that could easily be addressed in a private session but not in group Pilates reformer or mat classes. These clients had excess muscular tension in their chest and solar plexus and rib cage. Also their back muscles were pulled up towards their neck rather than resting down their spine. These issues caused them to look bent forward and to lose range of motion in their shoulder joints. Because of this lack of alignment teaching them abdominal work was difficult because it bothered their neck and lower back. I decided that in order to move people into a more advanced workout routine these issues needed to be addressed.

I began using the half foam roller in one of my group mat classes and after a few weeks started to notice big changes in my clients shoulder range of motion and less overall tension in their chest and stomach. Their posture was improving faster and their abdominal work was no longer bothering their neck. I became very enamored with the foam roller and have used it ever since.

## What Is Pilates?

Joseph Hubertus Pilates began inventing his body of work that he called Contrology around 1900. In is 60's around 1945 he published the book "Return to Life with Contrology" which outlined the philosophies and mat exercises behind what is now known as Pilates (puh- LAT-us) or (Pih-LAT-teez). Pilates is a series of whole body exercises coupled with specific breathing patterns. It is known for improving posture, increasing flexibility, connecting mind and body, improving circulation and joint health. Pilates has proven itself invaluable not only as a fitness endeavor, but also as an important adjunct to professional sports training and physical rehabilitation of all kinds.

## A Word on Posture

In my experience going from horrendous posture to regularly being complimented for my alignment, the best posture comes from releasing not straining to hold a position. In other words, you want to relax the body into a nice posture. I have heard too many times the misguided cues: Squeeze your belly button back and up, tuck your pelvis under and pull your shoulders back and down. I tried this approach for many years and have come to the conclusion that these types of cues cause more harm than good.

My approach is to teach the body how to release and *then* how to engage. If you are too focused on engagement first, you will continue to overly shorten the muscles on the front of the body, which will cause the back of the body to be overstretched.

The foam roller allows the body to open up and relax. I can exercise from a place where I am maximally released and tension is allowed to let go. Now of course, sometimes I lay on the foam roller and I am still holding tension. That is normal. It will begin to release over time.

At the end of this book I will discuss standing and give you cues that allow you to release into great posture.

## What If Laying on the Foam Roller Hurts?

It is normal to have discomfort when first lying on a foam roller especially if your back is very tight. If this is the case, I recommend taking time to lie on the floor without a foam roller with your knees bent for 10 minutes twice a day for a couple of weeks to reduce your tension. Then try just lying on the foam roller doing no exercises for 10 minutes a day for 2 weeks. Work up slowly to doing just 1 or 2 of the beginning arm warm ups. Generally, people start to find the foam roller more comfortable and even begin to love it!! If that doesn't work then you might need some help releasing your muscles and fascia: Alexander Technique, Feldenkrais, Rolfing, Massage, Cranial Sacral, Shiatsu, to name a few techniques that I have used to loosen up.

Most importantly, *don't give up* lying on a foam roller was initially uncomfortable for me. Now my back craves it and so many of my students over the past 15 years have had the same experience. While you explore your options, be safe. If you have osteoporosis ask your doctor if using a foam roller is safe for you. If you are experiencing muscle spasms and sharp pains, lie on the floor on your back with knees bent and a stack of magazines about the height of your hand under your head and let your back release. This is called the Constructive Rest Position in Alexander Technique. If all is well, let's get started.

## What You Need

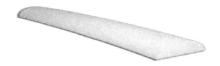

**6"x 36" High-Density Half Foam Roller**

**2, 3, or 5 lb. Hand Weights**

The 6"x 36" high-density half foam roller can be ordered online on Amazon or many other sites on the Internet. Expect shipping costs to be a little high because it is large and therefore expensive to ship. This course is designed for the half foam roller and not the full-size foam roller, so, be careful when you are ordering to order the right one. The full-size round foam rollers are a little too big for what we are doing and won't feel comfortable. Also, they are difficult to stabilize and you will run into the problem of them slipping out from under you.

The free-weights you need depend on your flexibility and strength. If your rotator cuff/shoulder joint has full Range of Motion and you are strong then you should use a 5 lbs. weight. If your rotator cuff or your shoulder joint is a little bit tight but you are strong then I'd recommend 3 lbs. weights. If your shoulders are a little tight and your muscles are a bit weaker then I'd go with 2 lbs. If your rotator cuff has very limited range of motion, I would recommend no weights and focusing on your flexibility instead.

## Audio Version

If you would prefer to listen to this routine as a flowing workout, go to: **http://www.intuitpilates.com/easypilatesworkout**

# CHAPTER 1
# GETTING STARTED ON THE FOAM ROLLER

## Alignment

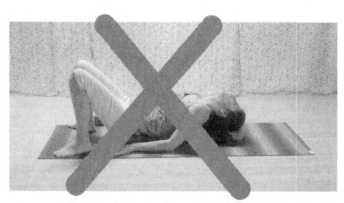

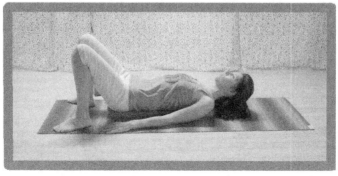

**Cues:**
- Shoulders should rest open and be relaxed into the foam roller.
- Tummy should be soft and relaxed.
- There should be a small space between your lower back (lumbar part of the spine) and the foam roller.
- Your tailbone area (sacrum) should be rest into the foam roller. Chin and forehead should be on the same plane.

**Imagery:**
- Imagine you are lying on a grassy slope with your head going down hill and your feet at the top of the hill.
- Imagine there is a heavy ball resting underneath your sternum in between your ribs.

# Abdominal Engagement

I will use the term "engage your abdominals" throughout this book so I want to give you a brief description of what I mean. Abdominal engagement is definitely an art and it has taken me many years to perfect it and it takes my clients years to perfect it. I will not be able to do an in-depth study on the art of abdominal engagement here but I will give you a brief synopsis.

First, you want abdominal engagement to be based on lengthening not shortening. So allow the spine to stay long, keep your tailbone down and the back of the neck long. Then, engage your ribs towards each other as you exhale. Sometimes, making the shhhhhhh (with the force of shushing someone across a crowded room) sound as you exhale can be helpful to allow you to feel this engagement. Next, draw your navel back towards your spine without flattening your lumbar curve. Finally, imagine making the muscles between your two hip bones/iliac crests form a smile.

I know, I know; this is a lot to consider. Abdominal engagement is not easy to teach and its not easy to learn but just take it one step at a time and hopefully I will get around to making a video series on it!

# CHAPTER 2
# SHOULDER WARM-UPS

(These are designed to be a warm-up so do as many as you like. Also, once the shoulders are warm all of these can be done with free-weights)

## Back Stroke

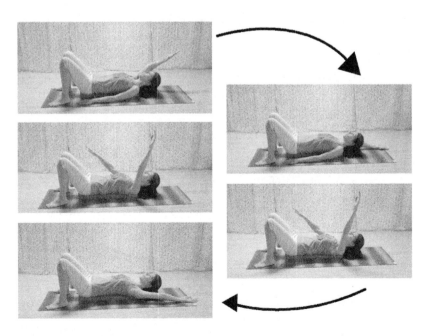

**Cues:**

- Start with both palms facing down next to your hips.
- Leaving the left arm lying next to you, raise your right arm off the floor and keeping the elbow straight bring it over head flat on the floor.
- Bring your left arm to overhead and the right arm back to the start position.
- Continue switching.
- The shoulder blades should melt into the foam roller.
- The muscles between the shoulder blades should be getting a massage.
- Keep the elbows straight.
- Repeat 8-10 x's.

**Note:** If the elbows cannot stay straight when the arm is overhead it is an indication that the rotator cuff is tight.

## Hug-a-Tree

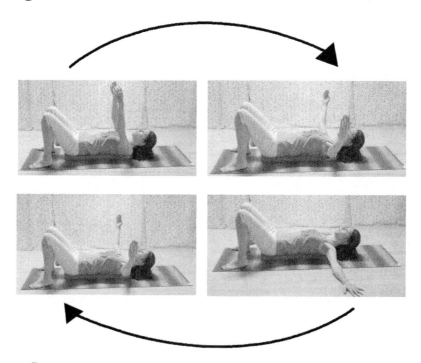

**Cues:**

- Start by extending both arms toward the ceiling out in front of your chest palms facing each other.

- Soften the elbows so they are slightly bent and relax the shoulder blades around the foam roller.
- Open the arms imagining that the collarbone is wrapping around the foam roller until your elbows touch the floor.
- Again keep the shoulder blades heavily weighted into the foam roller. Lead the movement with the upper arm bone. At the bottom of the movement stretch the chest muscles by flipping the palms facing down and reaching the arms long.
- Bring the hands back towards the ceiling making sure to soften the elbows again and bring the arms back over the chest palms facing each other.
- Repeat 8-10 x's.

## Angel Arms

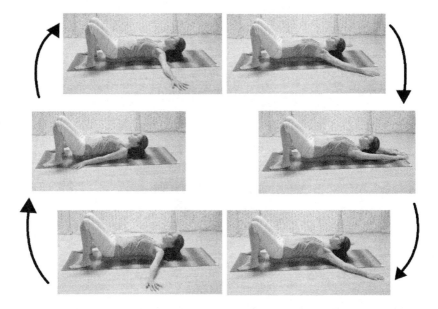

**Cues:**
- Start with both palms facing down next to your hips.
- Keep them on the floor and slide as high as you can as if doing a snow angel.
- Don't flip the palms towards the ceiling until you can no longer raise your arms without lifting them off the floor.

- Flip the palms towards the ceiling and continue until your arms are overhead.
- As you begin to slide them back down towards your hips flip the palms back towards the floor as soon as you comfortably can.
- Make sure your shoulder blades stay relaxed around the foam roller throughout the movement.
- Repeat 8 x's.

## Rotator Cuff Opener

(Rotator Cuff Definition: The rotator cuff is a group of muscles and tendons that surround the shoulder joint, keeping the head of your upper arm bone firmly within the shallow socket of the shoulder.)

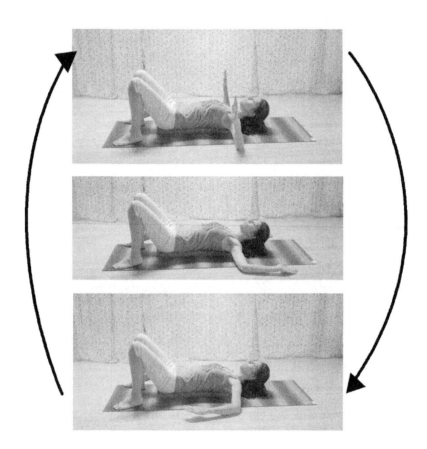

**Cues:**

- Start with both elbows planted on the floor at shoulder height elbows bent and fingertips toward the ceiling, palms facing the feet.
- Keeping your elbows on the floor, wind your upper arm bones forward until your forearms, wrists and hands are touching the floor. If you can't touch the floor go as far as you can go.
- Wind back to the start point.
- Then rotate the upper arm bones so that the top of the forearms, wrists and hands touch the floor.
- Focus on keeping the shoulder blades resting into the foam roller.
- Repeat 8 x's.

# Alternating Rotator Cuff Opener

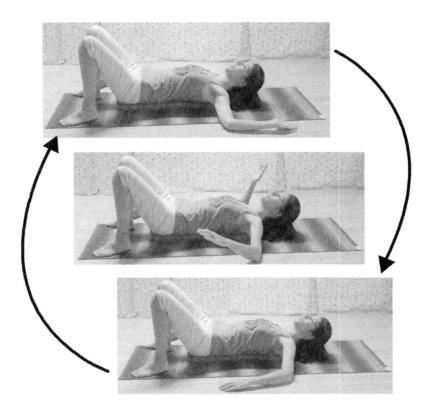

**Cues:**

- Start with both elbows planted on the floor at shoulder height elbows bent, fingertips toward the ceiling, palms facing feet.
- Keeping your elbows in the same spot rotate your right arm forward and your left arm backward ending with both wrists and hands touching the floor.
- Continue alternating one arm forward and the other arm backward.
- Feel as though you are melting tension in the chest muscles in order to increase the range of motion in the rotator cuff.
- Repeat 8 x's.

# CHAPTER 3
# WEIGHTED ARM SERIES

(Grab your free weights, unless your range of motion is very limited; if so, just do these movements without free weights and focus on flexibility over strength.)

## Chest Press

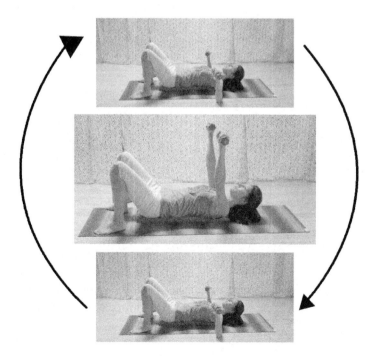

**Cues:**

- Grab your free weights and plant your elbows on the floor at shoulder height with your forearm perpendicular to the floor, palms facing your feet.
- Keeping your shoulder blades wrapped around the foam roller extend your elbows towards the ceiling.
- Bend the elbows and return to your start position.
- The shoulders should stay relaxed and open throughout the movement.
- Repeat 8-20 x's.

## Pec Stretch

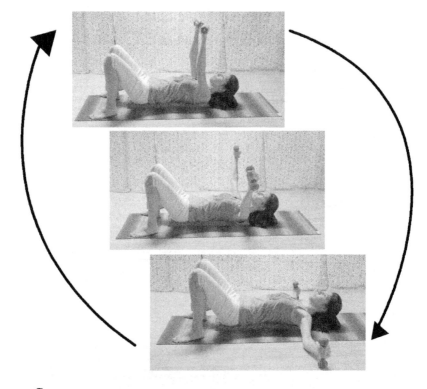

**Cues:**

- Start with your arms outstretched above your chest, hands holding weights toward the ceiling, palms facing your feet.
- Open your arms straight out to the side at shoulder height. Once touching the floor, focus on stretching your pectoralis/chest muscles.

- Bring the arms back up to center keeping your shoulder blades resting into the foam roller.
- Repeat 8-20 x's.

## Overhead to Hip

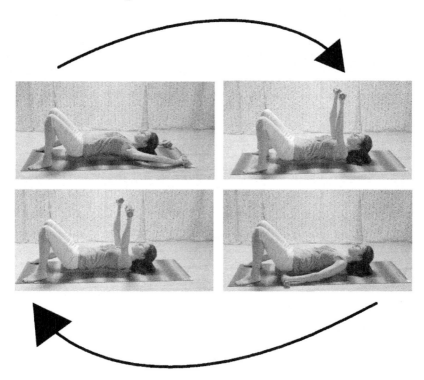

**Cues:**

- Engage your abdominal muscles to protect your rotator cuff by squeezing your rib cage towards the centerline of your body. (See "Abdominal Engagement" Chapter One)
- Holding your free weights, palms facing feet, start with both arms over chest toward the ceiling. Carefully bring them overhead and rest them on the floor.
- Keeping the abdominal engagement, bring the free weights back over your chest and continue until your hands are resting next to your hips on the floor.
- Repeat 8-20 x's.

# Backstroke with Weights

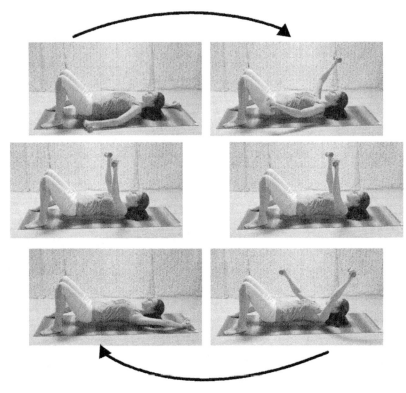

**Cues:**

- Start with both arms extended over chest straight up to the ceiling, shoulder blades resting around the foam roller and abdominal muscles engaged by drawing the ribs towards the centerline of the body.
- Bring your right arm to rest overhead on the floor and the left arm to rest on the floor next to your hips.
- Switch the positions of your arms as though doing the backstroke.
- Continue to engage your abdominals all the while resting your scapula on the foam roller.
- Repeat 8-20 x's.

## Hug-a-Tree Palms Out

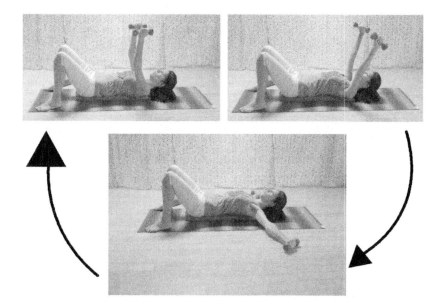

**Cues:**

- Start with both arms over chest toward the ceiling, palms facing each other, scapula rested against the foam roller.
- Rotate the palms facing out while opening the arms to the floor.
- Luxuriate in a chest stretch then rotate the palms facing the ceiling and return to arms over chest.
- Repeat 8-20 x's.

# Bicep Curl

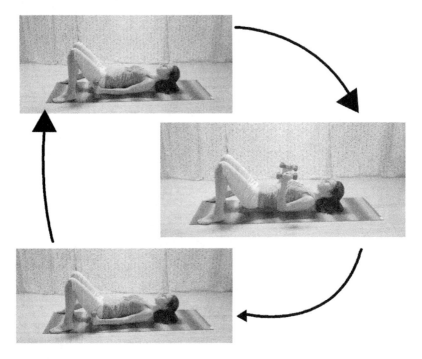

**Cues:**

- Start with both arms on the floor down by your hips. With your palms facing your hips holding the free weights.
- Keep your elbows on the floor and bend your elbows and extend back to the floor.
- Focus on your biceps and keep your shoulder from rounding forward and relax the scapula around the foam roller.
- Repeat 8-24 x's.

# Weighted Rotator Cuff

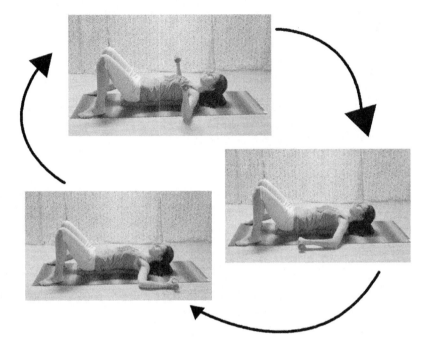

### Cues:

- Start with upper arms lying flat shoulder height on the floor and forearms upright facing your feet.
- Keeping elbows on the floor rotate the upper arm bones forward and bring weights to the floor.
- Rotate the upper arm bones backward using the elbows as a fulcrum point and bring the weights to the floor above your head.
- Make sure your chest stays as open and relaxed as possible.
- Repeat 8-20 x's. (Follow up with Alternating Rotator Cuff).

## Small Arm Circles

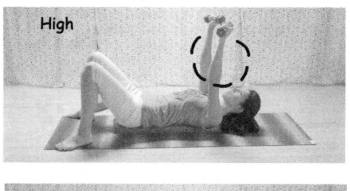

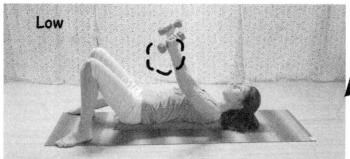

**Cues:**

- Start with the arms outstretched over your chest towards the ceiling at shoulder height.
- Make small circles on the ceiling with your free weights first rotating clockwise 8 x's and then rotating counter clockwise 8 x's.
- Feel the movement happening in the shoulder joint and not in the neck or chest.
- And of course, keep the scapula resting on the foam roller!
- For a little more challenge, lower the arms toward your feet and do the same clockwise 8 x's and counter clockwise circles 8 x's.
- If you are able to keep your chest relaxed and open, you can lower the free weights to just above the floor.

# CHAPTER FOUR
# LEG AND FOOTWORK

## Flex and Point

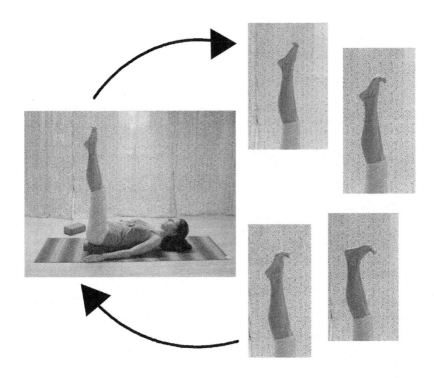

**Cues:**

- Keeping your tailbone weighted into the foam roller extend your legs straight up to the ceiling. (If you find it difficult to hold both legs up just do 1 leg at a time)
- Notice when you fully extend your legs to straight how the front of your thighs must work.
- Starting with your feet pointed, bring your toes back towards your knees (it will look like a Barbie doll foot)
- Then keeping your toes pulled back towards your knees flex your ankle joint bringing the entire foot back towards the knee. At this point you will feel the top of the feet and front of the shins working and the calves stretching.
- While keeping the toes flexed back toward your knees (Barbie doll feet), point your ankle joint forward.
- Lastly, round the toes so that your entire foot is pointed.
- Repeat 8-10x's.

## Straddle Stretches

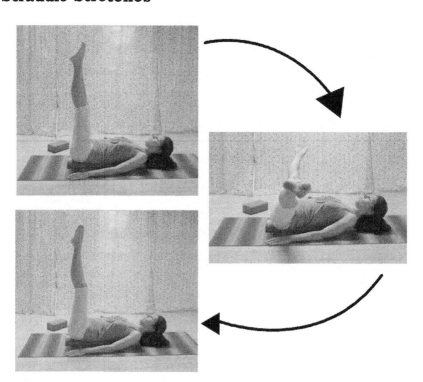

**Cues:**

- Keeping your tailbone weighted into the foam roller, extend your legs to the ceiling. Point toes toward the ceiling.
- Rotate from the hip joints so that the backs of knees are together and your thighs are turned out.
- Open each leg out to side as far as you are comfortable.
- Keeping the legs turned out draw the legs back together slowly as though you are zipping up a zipper from the inner thighs to the heels.
- Repeat 8-10x's.

# Hip Opener

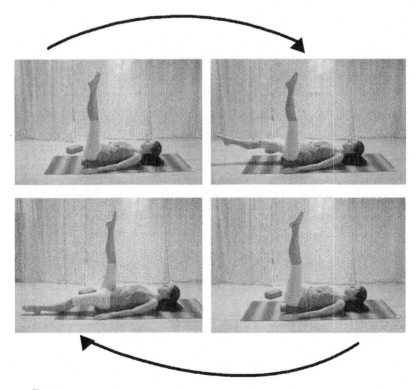

**Cues:**

- Keeping your tailbone weighted into the foam roller extend both legs to the ceiling.
- Initiating the movement from the front of the hip while keeping the abdominal muscles engaged and while keeping the left leg extended, lower your right leg down

as far as you can toward the floor position you started in.

- Bring the right leg back up to point towards the ceiling initiating from the front of the hip and lower the other leg to the floor.
- Repeat 10-12x's.

## Ceiling Plies

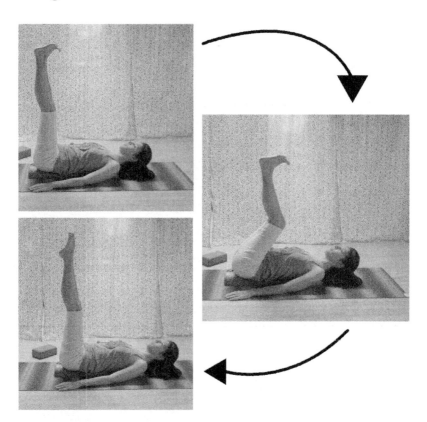

**Cues:**
- Keeping your tailbone weighted into the foam roller, extend your legs to the ceiling.
- Flex both toes and ankles.
- While keeping your heels facing the ceiling not the front wall fold the hip joint as far as you can while keeping the tailbone on the foam roller. Bend the knees.
- Extend your legs and point your ankles and toes.

- Continue to extend the legs fully until your hamstrings (back of thighs) feel a stretch and your quadriceps (front of thighs) feel engaged.
- Repeat 8-10x's.

# CHAPTER 5
# AB SERIES

(Rotate the foam roller horizontally and place under the tips of your shoulder blades. For women right at the bra line)

## Small Contraction

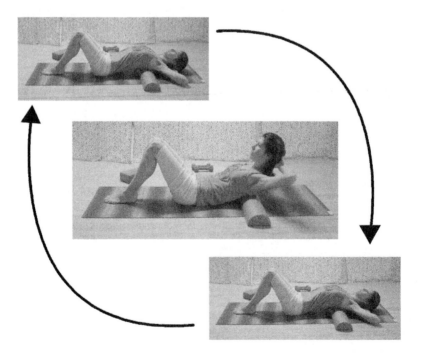

**Cues:**
- With the foam roller under the tip of the scapula, bend your knees and with your feet on the mat, keep the ankles, knees and inner thighs pressing toward each other.
- Inhale and lengthen the front of your body and wrap the upper back over the foam roller.
- Keep the chin and forehead on the same plane and keep the back of the neck long. Hands behind your head.
- Exhale and contract the upper ribs together to initiate a contraction in the abdominals that will lift the head off the floor. (Do not initiate the contraction with the neck. Instead, initiate the contraction by drawing the ribs towards each other.)
- Repeat 8-10x's.

## Table Top Contraction

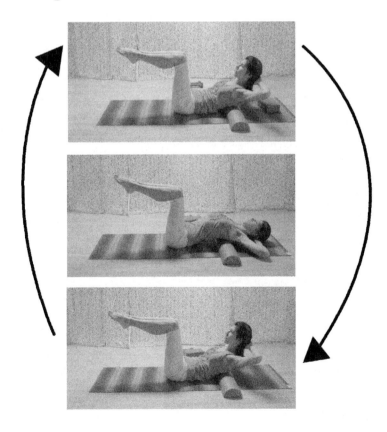

**Cues:**

- Starting with the foam roller under the tip of the scapula, bring your legs into a table-top position meaning there is a 90 degree angle at the hip joints and at the knee joint. (If you find this difficult on your lower back bring your knees closer to your chest) Your lower leg will be parallel to the floor.
- Inhale and lengthen the front of your body and wrap the upper back over the foam roller. Hands behind your head.
- Keep the chin and forehead on the same plane and keep the back of the neck long.
- Exhale and contract the upper ribs together to initiate a contraction in the abdominals that will lift the head off the floor. (Do not initiate the contraction with the neck. Instead, initiate the contraction by drawing the ribs towards each other.)
- Repeat 8-10x's.

## Roll-Up

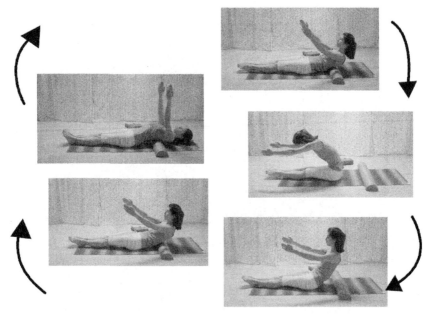

**Cues:**

- Start with your legs outstretched on the mat with ankles, knees, and inner thighs touching, toes pointed and arms extended straight up over chest, palms facing each other and your head and back extended over the foam roller onto the floor.

- Inhale in place and exhale. Draw the ribs together and curl up lifting your head, neck and upper back only to the bottom of your scapula.
- Using a full breath continue to roll up one vertebra at a time until you are on your sitz bones holding your tummy into a contraction, arms reaching forward towards your feet.
- On a full inhale begin to exhale slowly and roll back down one vertebra at a time until your scapula reaches the foam roller.
- Inhale and open the front of the body exhale and wrap the upper back over the foam roller and rest the head back on the mat.
- Repeat 3-5x's.

## Single Leg Stretch

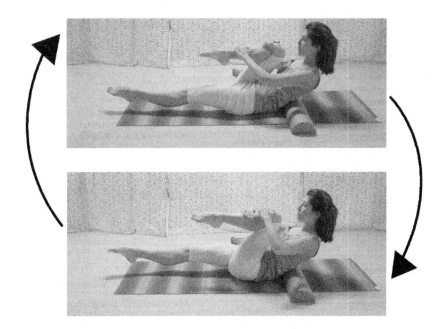

**Cues:**
- Start in a small contraction with scapula resting on the foam roller upper back and head off the mat. Bring your right knee to your chest and extend your left leg so that it's hovering a few inches over the mat.

- Inhale while you switch your legs by bringing the left leg back towards the chest and the right leg extended over the mat.
- Exhale while you switch again.
- Repeat this pattern 8-16x's

## Single Leg Lower

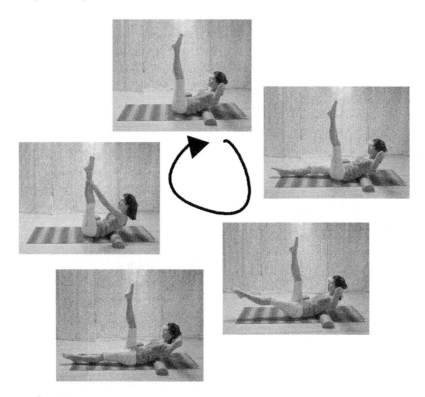

**Cues:**

- Bring your hands behind your head and support your neck during this exercise.
- Keeping your tailbone weighted into the mat, extend your legs to the ceiling and curl your head up off the mat and scapula touching the foam roller.
- While your other leg stays stationary inhale and lower your right leg to the mat.
- Exhale and bring your right leg back up and lower your left.
- Alternate the two positions 8-16x's.

- Reach up and hold onto both of your shins. (This is your rest position should you get tired during this exercise.)

## Double Leg Lower

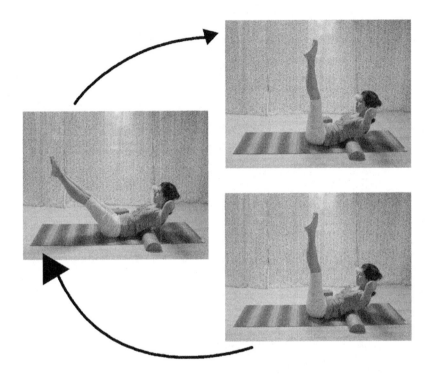

### Cues:
- Keeping your tailbone weighted into the mat, extend your legs to the ceiling, head curled off the mat and scapula touching the foam roller. Hands are behind the head supporting the neck.
- Inhale in place. Opening the front of the hips exhale and lower both legs towards the mat. Only go as low as you can go while keeping the belly button pulled towards your spine.
- Inhale with the legs low. Exhale bring both legs back up towards the ceiling.
- Repeat 8-10x's.
- If your back feels tired, skip this exercise.

# CHAPTER 6
# SIDE-LYING SERIES

(Roll over onto your side and place the foam roller just below the armpit on the bra line.  Knees will be stacked on top of each other at a 90-degree angle.)

## Shoulder Circumlocution

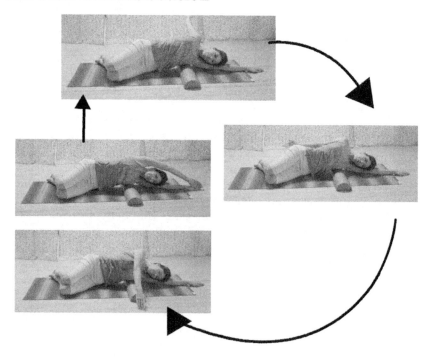

**Cues:**
- Start with both arms stretched overhead.
- Make sure throughout the movement that you are keeping space between the bottom of the ear and the shoulder.
- Bring the shoulder through its full range of motion as you move your top arm circle it behind you towards the back wall, to the hip, in front of the chest and back to overhead.
- Repeat 8-10x's.
- Repeat lying on the other side.

## Rotation

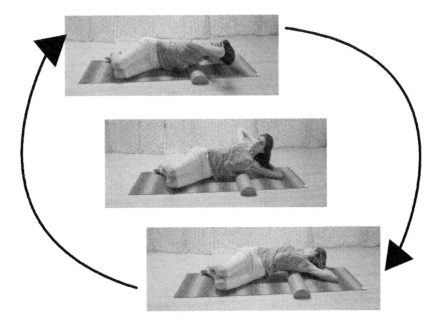

**Cues:**
- Keep knees stacked on top of each other at a 90-degree angle.
- Bring your hands behind your head and lie as flat on the floor as you can.
- Keeping the hips stacked on top of each other, inhale and keeping your pelvis still rotate the chest forward as far as your waistline can stretch. Even as far as facing the mat.
- Think of lengthening the front of the body throughout the movement.

- Return to center rotating from the waistline.
- Keeping your pelvis still open the chest towards the ceiling.
- Repeat 8-12 x's.
- Repeat with knees stacked to the other side.

# CHAPTER 7
# PSOAS STRETCHES

**A Word on the Psoas**

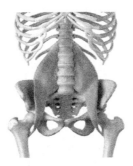

The psoas is the deepest layer of the core. In fact, it allows us to stand upright without destabilizing the lumbar spine/lower back. When we have poor posture often the muscles of the back become overstretched and weakened and the psoas gets short and tight. All of your intention in standing and during abdominal workouts should be in lengthening this muscle. The following exercises might prove challenging at first if your psoas is tight. These will help you to lengthen it back out which is crucial to having great posture.

# Swan

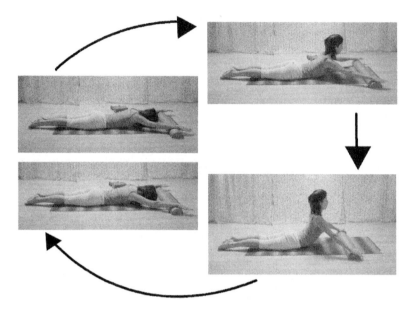

**Cues:**

- Lie in a prone position/on your tummy legs fully extended arms reaching overhead with your hands on the foam roller.
- Draw your rib cage together and lift your belly button up towards your chin.
- Keeping the back of your neck long (imagine holding an apple between your chin and chest) and your latissimus dorsi/ back muscle engaged (imagine bringing your shoulder blades towards your hips) lift your chest off the mat sliding the foam roller towards you.
- Keep lifting the belly button towards your chin and emphasize stretching the psoas muscles.
- Again keeping the back of the neck long and the belly button engaged towards the chin roll back down one vertebra at a time sliding the foam roller back to your start position.
- Repeat 3-5 x's

## Hip Stretch

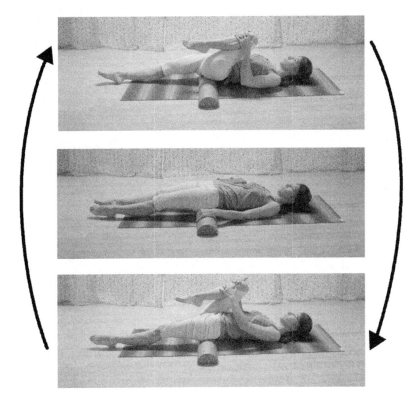

**Cues:**
- While laying supine/on your back on the mat, place the foam roller horizontally under your sacrum.
- Bring one knee back towards your chest and fully extend the other leg out on the mat. Hold the stretch for 1 minute.
- Switch legs. Hold the stretch for 1 minute.
- If desired repeat on both sides.

# Corpse Pose

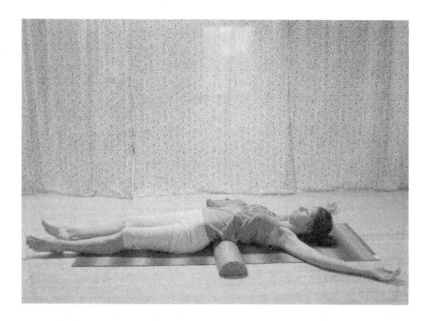

**Cues:**

- While lying supine on the mat, place the foam roller under your lumbar spine or behind the belly button.
- Your legs and arms can be spread out.
- Your tailbone should touch the floor.
- If this is painful, this is a sign that your psoas is very short. Consider bending your knees and tucking your pelvis so that your tailbone can be further away from the floor. Then slowly lower the pelvis incrementally until your back is used to the position. If it does not improve, do the corpse pose without the foam roller.

# CHAPTER 8
# WHERE TO GO FROM HERE

## Standing posture

Now that you've finished your exercises, it's time to stand up, which is the most important exercise you can do. Since we spend a majority of our lives standing and walking, what you do here is going to impact your posture the most. Exercising a couple of hours a week is nothing compared to the many hours you spend upright. First of all, I encourage you check out a video I made about standing posture. It's easier to see me show you what to do than to tell you. If you click on the link below I'll email it to you. It will show you typical posture pitfalls and give you some guidelines on how not to fall into them.

**If you would like me to email you a video on postural strategies go to this link and send me your email:**

**http://www.intuitpilates.com/freevideo**

After you watch the video, here are a few ideas that can help you improve your posture.

**#1. Notice:**
You have to be able to know where you are in order to know where you want to go.

Start with the head and neck. Stand in front of a mirror and assess how the head is resting on the neck. Notice if the neck looks even on both sides, or if one side is shorter than the other. Does it pull forward like a turtle? Does it shorten in the back? Just notice what it's doing.

Next notice the shoulders. Do they round forward? Is one higher than the other? Are you holding them back? Are they pulled down towards the hips? Do they feel comfortable?

Become aware of your torso. Is the stomach gripped or relaxed? Do you feel anxious with butterflies in your stomach? Does your lower back feel compressed? Does your back hurt?

Move awareness to the pelvis? Are the buttocks muscles tight or released? Is the pelvis tilted forward, tilted back, or neutral?

Become aware of the legs. Are they gripped? Do they feel heavy? Do they feel light? Do you have pain in the knees?

Lastly, notice the feet. Is weight distributed towards the balls of the feet? Is weight distributed towards the heels? Do the arches touch the floor or is weight on the outside of the foot?

## #2. Release:
If the neck is being pulled forward, stop pulling the neck forward. If the neck is being pulled backward, stop pulling the neck backward.

If the breath is being held, stop holding the breath.

If the legs are gripping, relax the muscles of the legs.

If the buttocks and stomach are tight, let go of the tension.

Relax whatever tension is being held throughout the body.

## #3. Direct:
Directing the body and mind requires a clean slate or a body free from tension. Then we are able to start to get specific about alignment.

Start with the head and neck. Keeping the neck free (not fixed or gripped) allow the back of your neck to lengthen.

Next allow your ribs to be free and floating and your breathing is to be easy and not labored or held.

From there the shoulders should relax, as though resting on the free ribs.

The abdominal muscles should be relaxed and open. Allow the upper half of your torso (the ribs) to gently rise towards the head of the body and the lower half of the torso to release towards the tail of the body.

Ensure that the buttocks are not gripping and the tailbone is not tucked between the legs.

Keep space between the pelvis and the lower ribs to ensure that the lumbar spine is not overly arched.

Lastly, keep your feet evenly weighted between the center of the heel bone, the ball of the big toe and the ball of the pinky toe. (You can test this by lifting your toes off the floor while keeping the heels and balls of the foot on the floor. If you sway backwards then you are not evenly weighted. If you lift the toes and the rest of the body is unaffected then you are evenly weighted.)

**Don't Forget:**
If you would prefer to listen to this routine as a flowing workout, go to: **http://www.intuitpilates.com/easypilatesworkout**

**Gratitude:**
Thank you so much for buying and reading this book. It means a great deal to me. Teaching movement is my sacred work while I'm here on the planet. After having children and taking a break from teaching, I learned that I'm not a teacher unless I have students. So, I have tons of gratitude for everyone who listens and learns from me.

Also, the body constantly changes and presents new obstacles for us all myself included. There have been times that I needed intense workouts and times that I enjoyed more subtle routines, times that I've taken breaks and times that I go full force. Remember to listen to your body. I always let my body, my enthusiasm, my passions be my guide. If you are feeling defeated by any routine get it out of your life. To keep learning and growing in your movement find something that lights you up, feels encouraging and inspires you.

Lastly, I want to thank all of my teachers, who have challenged me to grow. I want to thank my husband for watching T.V. alone while I write. I want to thank my clients without your support I could not continue on this path. Lastly, I want to thank my boys who gave me the courage to move my studio home, which has inspired me to be creative and develop my own work. My heart is very full.

If you have questions or concerns feel free to email me at KristenFryer@IntuitPilates.com.

# ABOUT THE AUTHOR

Helping people find their way to the body and life that they deserve is my greatest joy. Thank you for giving me a chance to help you.

I'm told that this is the part where I show you why I'm qualified. And why I think the techniques in this workout will move you toward the posture results that you want to see.

We could talk about the thousands of hours I've spent traveling the U.S. training with Ron Fletcher, Pat Guyton, or Kyria Sabin, and other founding leaders of the Pilates movement. (Not to mention the countless hours with Alexander Technique professionals) Or, I could share stories of victory from the hundreds of clients that I've been fortunate enough to create transformation with in my studio. But...

**The experience that has best prepared me to help you release pain and develop balance was what I learned from healing myself. I first learned about Alexander Technique, Pilates and Theta Healing to save my own life and livelihood.**

17 years ago I was a total mess. Still in college, completely bent over and wracked with pain. I checked myself into the hospital, only to be sent home with pills. No doctor could clearly explain what was wrong with me, much less how I was supposed to heal. This was the beginning of my life's work: finding the root of physical pain and stopping it at the source.

What began as a curse has become my greatest blessing and gift. Movement is how I communicate. Being active is the key to how I learn, play and teach. There is indescribable freedom and power in treating your body right.

Let's get there together.

Printed in Great Britain
by Amazon

42586721R00030